JOHN JUSTICE

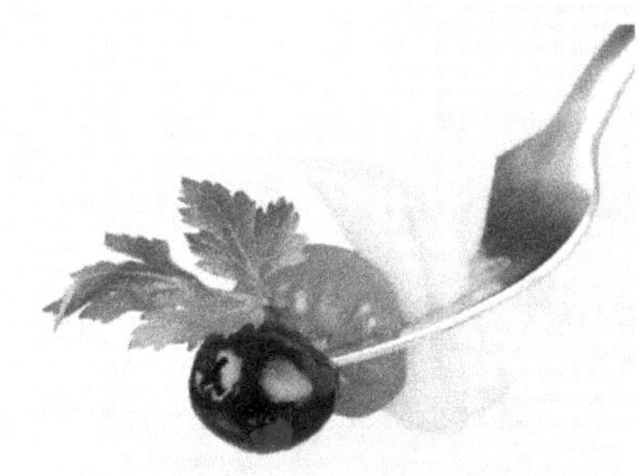

Healthy

Food Recipes For Diet

LIVING FOOD

A CONCISE BUT ULTIMATE GUIDE TO EATING LIVE FOOD TO A HEALTHIER AND CANCER FREE LIFE.

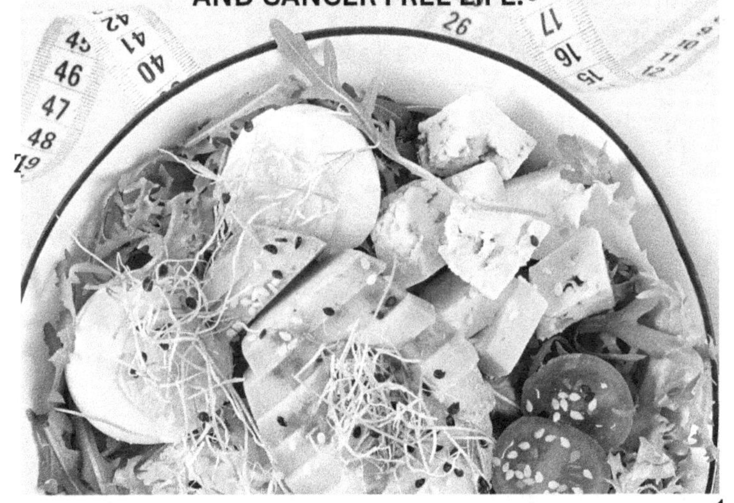

Table of Content

Chapter 1 Introduction

Step into a world where every meal is a vibrant journey, and each bite is a celebration of vitality. Living foods, the culinary artisans of nature, beckon you to savor the extraordinary. Imagine a banquet of raw, unadulterated goodness, where the essence of life bursts forth in a kaleidoscope of flavors. Here, the kitchen transforms into a sanctuary where fruits, vegetables, and sprouted wonders converge, creating a canvas of taste that transcends the ordinary. It's not just about sustenance; it's about embracing the aliveness of each ingredient, inviting you to partake in a sensory symphony that dances on your taste buds. Welcome to the realm of living foods—a realm where nutrition meets artistry, and every meal is a brushstroke painting the masterpiece of your well-being. Let the journey into this culinary wonderland commence, where the feast is not just on the table but is a celebration of life itself.

Definition of Living Food

Living food refers to raw, unprocessed, and uncooked edibles that retain their natural vitality and enzymatic activity. These foods are often plant-based, including raw fruits, vegetables, sprouts, and nuts. The concept revolves around consuming food in its most natural state, preserving essential nutrients, enzymes, and life force that proponents believe contribute to enhanced health and

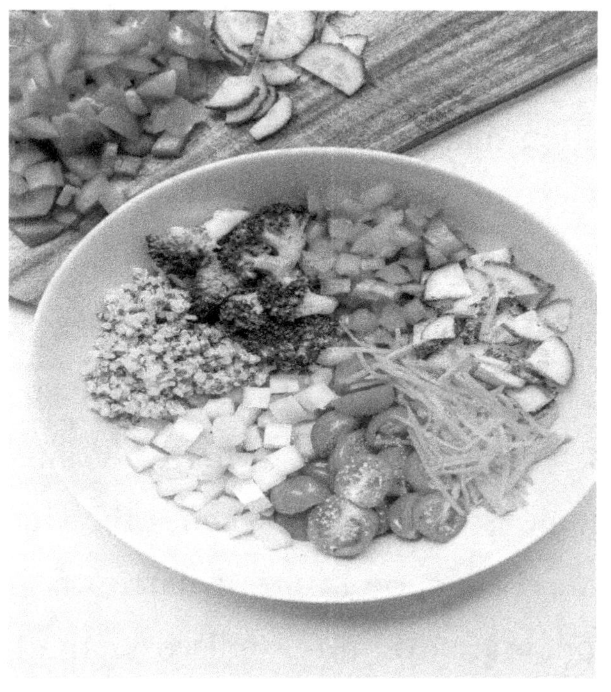

well-being. In essence, living foods are considered a dynamic source of nourishment, embracing the idea that unaltered, raw elements offer a more vibrant and holistic approach to nutrition.

These are not just meals; they are celebrations of nature's raw generosity. A definition that transcends the kitchen, living foods are a symphony of flavors, colors, and nutrients, delivering a feast for the senses and nourishment for the soul. With every bite, experience the living heartbeat of fruits, vegetables, and sprouted grains—a harmonious melody that echoes the vitality of the Earth on your palate. In this gastronomic adventure, rediscover the true meaning of nutrition, as living foods not only fuel the body but also awaken a zest for life in every delicious mouthful.

Historical Perspective

In the tapestry of time, the historical roots of living foods unfold like a cherished secret, whispered through centuries. Picture ancient civilizations, their culinary wisdom steeped in the raw essence of nature. Millennia ago, our ancestors cultivated an intimate dance with the Earth, savoring the untamed offerings it provided. From the vibrant markets of ancient Rome to the mystic gardens of Asia, the pages of history reveal a tapestry woven with the threads of living foods.

In the annals of time, luminaries and healers marveled at the life force inherent in uncooked, unaltered nourishment. The ancient Greeks, with their reverence for balance, embraced raw foods as an elixir for vitality. Across the Silk Road, Chinese sages extolled the virtues of living foods in harmonizing the body and spirit.

Fast forward to the Renaissance, where Leonardo da Vinci's sketches hinted at a fascination with the simplicity of uncooked fare. The historical panorama unveils visionaries and pioneers who, like culinary alchemists, recognized the transformative power of living foods on human well-being.

As we journey through epochs, from the rustic kitchens of medieval Europe to the enlightenment of the 19th century, the historical perspective of living foods reveals a nuanced narrative—one that whispers the timeless truth that nature's bounty, in its raw authenticity, has always been a tapestry woven with the threads of life and health.

Chapter 2 Nutritional Benefits

Enzymes and Bioavailability

Enzymes, those unsung maestros of the microscopic world, take center stage in the symphony of living foods. Picture a culinary ballet where every bite is choreographed by these molecular virtuosos. In the realm of living foods, these tiny powerhouses are not mere ingredients; they are alchemists that unlock the hidden treasures within each mouthful.

As you indulge in the crisp succulence of a fresh apple or savor the earthy crunch of a vibrant salad, know that you're not just tasting; you're partaking in an enzymatic sonata. These living foods boast a symphony of enzymes—biological wizards that orchestrate the transformation of nutrients into a ballet of bioavailability.

Envision this biochemical ballet: enzymes pirouetting through the digestive stage, unraveling the complexities of proteins, fats, and carbohydrates. In the enchanted realm of living foods, these enzymes become culinary conjurers, ensuring that every nutrient, every essence, is not just present but is offered in a form readily embraced by your body.

This is not just a gastronomic experience; it's a nutritional pas de deux where the bioavailability of living foods transcends the

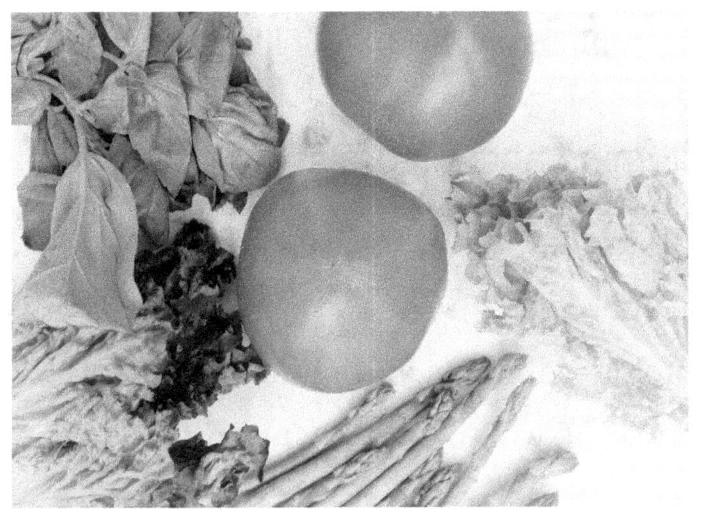

ordinary. Each enzymatic pirouette enhances the nutritional dance, ensuring that the nutrients are integrated seamlessly into your body's grand performance of health and vitality. In this gastronomic theater, living foods take a bow as the starring act, and enzymes—those invisible conductors—compose the melody of nourishment, making every bite a harmonious celebration of life.

Vitamins and Minerals

Within the vibrant tapestry of living foods, a kaleidoscope of nature's gifts unfolds—vitamins and minerals, the unsung heroes of well-being. Picture a feast where each color, each texture, tells a story of nutritional abundance.

In the kingdom of living foods, fruits, and vegetables are not mere culinary delights; they are nature's capsules, brimming with vitamins that sparkle like jewels in the crown of health. Bite into the crisp embrace of an orange, and you ingest a burst of vitamin C—a citrus symphony to fortify your immune realm. Delve into the verdant allure of spinach, and the whisper of vitamin K beckons, guiding your body in the dance of coagulation and bone health.

Yet, the banquet of living foods is not merely a vitaminic affair; it's a mineral-rich ballad, where nutrients like calcium, magnesium, and potassium waltz through the body, fortifying its foundations. In the crucible of nature's kitchen, minerals become the architects of bone strength, nerve function, and electrolyte balance.

Picture this: each bite of living foods, a harmonious medley of vitamins and minerals, weaving a nutritional sonnet that resonates within your very core. As you savor the symphony of colors on your plate, know that you're not just dining; you're partaking in a nutritional masterpiece where vitamins and minerals are the brushstrokes that paint the canvas of your holistic well-being.

Chapter 3 Types of Living Food

Raw Fruits and Vegetables

In the theater of nutrition, raw fruits and vegetables take center stage, each one a vibrant character in the unfolding drama of well-being. Picture the sun-kissed glow of an apple, and the verdant majesty of a cucumber—their raw, unaltered essence pulsating with life.

These raw gems aren't just ingredients; they are the very heartbeat of living foods, a gastronomic ballet where nature's bounty is celebrated in its pristine form. Bite into the crisp embrace of an uncooked carrot, and you're tasting the vitality of the earth, untamed and pure. Peel back the layers of a raw mango, and you're indulging in a sensory feast, where every fiber hums with the living energy of the sun and soil.

It's a culinary adventure where raw fruits and vegetables aren't just consumed; they're experienced. Picture the juiciness of a ripe watermelon, a symphony of hydration that quenches your thirst and replenishes your body's reservoirs. Envision the crunch of raw bell pepper, a vibrant explosion of colors and textures that titillate your taste buds.

In this gastronomic narrative, raw fruits and vegetables are not passive players—they are the protagonists, the guardians of vitamins, minerals, and antioxidants. As you partake in this living food spectacle, you're not just nourishing your body; you're becoming part of the epic tale where each raw bite is a tribute to the untamed beauty of nature's bounty, a celebration of life on your plate.

Sprouts and microgreens

Sprouts and microgreens, the verdant jewels of the living food kingdom, beckon us into a miniature cosmos of nutrition and flavor. Let's embark on an exhaustive exploration of these tiny powerhouses that pack a punch far beyond their size.

Birth of Vitality

Sprouts and microgreens are the embryonic stages of plants, bursting forth with life and nutritional abundance.

This early growth phase infuses them with concentrated nutrients, making them nutritional dynamos.

Sprouting Alchemy

The sprouting process unlocks dormant nutrients and enzymes, transforming seeds into vibrant, living foods.

Enzymes become catalysts for nutrient release, enhancing digestibility and bioavailability.

Microgreens Unveiled

Microgreens, the younger siblings of mature plants, offer a kaleidoscope of flavors, textures, and colors.

Despite their small stature, microgreens boast nutrient concentrations often higher than their mature counterparts.

Nutritional Bounty

Sprouts are nutritional powerhouses, rich in vitamins (A, C, K), minerals (iron, potassium), and protein.

Microgreens elevate the nutritional content further, packing antioxidants and phytonutrients in every leaf.

Culinary Symphony

Sprouts add a crisp, fresh crunch to salads and sandwiches, enhancing both taste and nutrition.

Microgreens, with their delicate flavors, elevate dishes as edible garnishes or as standalone salad greens.

DIY Cultivation

Sprouting at home is an accessible and cost-effective way to incorporate living foods into your diet.

Microgreens thrive in small spaces, making them ideal for urban dwellers to cultivate on windowsills or countertops.

Health Benefits

Both sprouts and microgreens are lauded for their potential to support digestion, boost immunity, and provide a natural energy kick.

Antioxidants present in these living foods contribute to cellular health and may have anti-inflammatory properties.

Caution and Considerations

While sprouts are generally safe, there's a risk of bacterial contamination, emphasizing the importance of proper hygiene during cultivation.

Microgreens, being delicate, require attention to avoid spoilage.

Culinary Innovation

Chefs worldwide embrace sprouts and microgreens for their versatility, using them to adorn dishes and infuse them with freshness.

The culinary world continually explores innovative ways to incorporate these living foods into various cuisines.

Closing the Loop

Sprouts and microgreens embody a full-circle narrative—from tiny seeds to nutritional powerhouses, and finally, to plates brimming with vitality.

Their journey encapsulates the essence of living foods, offering a delicious and nutrient-dense testament to the wonders of early plant life.

In the grand tapestry of living foods, sprouts, and microgreens stand as a testament to the profound nutritional potential that emerges from the tiniest of beginnings. From a culinary perspective, they are not just ingredients but living canvases that paint a vibrant picture of health and gastronomic delight.

Embark on a rich journey into the world of fermented foods, a culinary realm where microbes transform ingredients into a symphony of flavors, textures, and enhanced nutrition.

Fermentation Magic

Fermentation is a natural, ancient process where microorganisms—bacteria, yeast, or molds—metamorphose food components. This transformative dance unlocks new flavors, preserves food, and enhances its nutritional profile.

<u>Probiotic Powerhouse</u>
Fermented foods are renowned for their probiotic content, promoting a healthy balance of gut bacteria.

Probiotics contribute to digestive health, and immune function, and may even impact mental well-being.

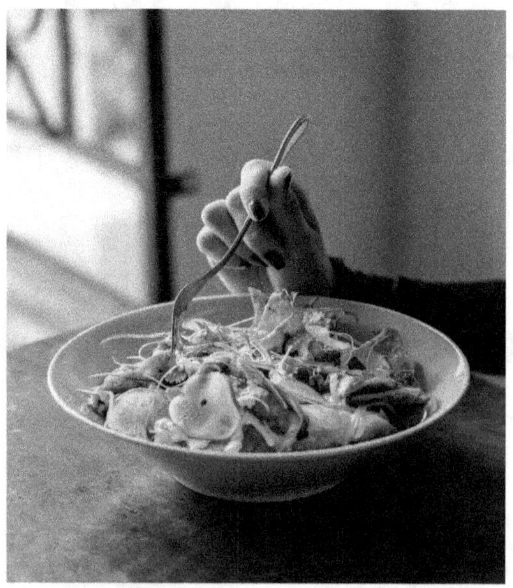

<u>Diverse Delicacies</u>

Explore a diverse range of fermented delights, from sauerkraut and kimchi to miso and tempeh.

Each culture brings forth unique fermentation traditions, yielding distinct textures and tastes.

Nutrient Amplification:
Fermentation unlocks nutrients, making them more bioavailable and easier for the body to absorb.
B vitamins, minerals, and certain amino acids may see an increase during the fermentation process.

Culinary Alchemy
Fermented foods add complexity and depth to culinary creations, from tangy pickles enhancing sandwiches to the umami richness of soy sauce.

Chefs globally embrace fermented ingredients for their ability to elevate dishes.

The Art of Pickling

Pickled vegetables, a subset of fermented foods, showcase the art of preserving seasonal harvests.

The tangy crunch of pickles and the versatility of pickled vegetables enhance a variety of dishes.

Brewing Traditions

Fermentation extends beyond solid foods to the realm of beverages, including kombucha, kefir, and traditional fermented teas.

These effervescent brews offer a refreshing alternative while delivering probiotic benefits.

Preservation Wisdom

Before refrigeration, fermentation was a crucial preservation method, allowing communities to store food for extended periods.

This ancient wisdom is still relevant today, contributing to both flavor and food security.

Health Impacts

Beyond gut health, fermented foods may have anti-inflammatory properties and could play a role in managing conditions like lactose intolerance.

Research explores the potential links between fermented foods and mental health.

DIY Fermentation

Engage in the art of home fermentation, from crafting your sauerkraut to experimenting with kombucha flavors.

DIY fermentation fosters a connection to traditional culinary practices and allows customization of flavors.

Caution and Considerations

While fermented foods offer numerous benefits, moderation is key.

Individuals with certain health conditions may need to exercise caution, and those new to probiotics should introduce them gradually.

<u>Cultural Significance</u>

Fermented foods often hold cultural significance, with recipes passed down through generations.

They reflect the ingenuity of communities in harnessing microbial transformations for culinary excellence.

In the grand saga of living foods, fermented delights stand as both culinary marvels and nutritional powerhouses. From the alchemy of bubbling brews to the tang of pickled perfection, fermented foods embody a tradition that transcends time, enriching our palates and fostering well-being through the captivating dance of microbes and ingredients.

Chapter 4 Health Impact

Improved Digestion

Embark on a comprehensive exploration of the digestive benefits bestowed by the consumption of living foods, unveiling the intricate interplay between these vibrant edibles and the intricate landscape of the digestive system.

Enzymatic Symphony

Living foods are a rich source of enzymes, the biochemical maestros that orchestrate the breakdown of nutrients.

Enzymes in raw fruits, vegetables, and sprouts enhance the digestive process, aiding in the efficient absorption of nutrients.

Bioavailability Boost

Raw and living foods retain their original nutritional integrity, ensuring that vital nutrients such as vitamins, minerals, and phytonutrients are readily available for absorption.

This enhanced bioavailability contributes to the nourishment of the body on a cellular level.

Fiber Fortification

Living foods, particularly fruits and vegetables, are abundant in dietary fiber.

Fiber promotes healthy digestion by adding bulk to stools, facilitating bowel regularity, and supporting a balanced gut microbiome.

Gut Microbiome Harmony
Probiotics present in fermented living foods foster a harmonious gut microbiome.
A balanced microbiome contributes to optimal digestion, and nutrient absorption, and may play a role in overall immune function.

Alleviation of Digestive Issues
The consumption of living foods has been associated with a reduction in common digestive issues, such as bloating, gas, and indigestion.

Enzymes and probiotics in these foods may aid in breaking down complex carbohydrates and supporting gut health.

pH Balance and Enzyme Activity

Living foods contribute to maintaining an optimal pH balance in the digestive tract. Enzymes function optimally within specific pH ranges, and a balanced environment supports their activity in breaking down food components.

Anti-Inflammatory Potential

Certain living foods, particularly those rich in antioxidants, may have anti-inflammatory properties.

Reduced inflammation in the digestive system can contribute to a more comfortable and efficient digestive process.

Satiety and Mindful Eating

The high water and fiber content in many living foods contributes to a feeling of satiety.

Mindful eating of living foods encourages a slower pace, aiding digestion and promoting a healthier relationship with food.

Hydration and Digestive Fluids

Living foods, with their inherent water content, contribute to hydration, a crucial factor in maintaining the fluidity of digestive processes.

Well-hydrated digestive fluids support the breakdown and absorption of nutrients.

Support for Digestive Organs

The nutrients and compounds in living foods may provide support for digestive organs such as the liver and pancreas. Antioxidants in these foods contribute to the protection of cells and tissues within the digestive system.

Culinary Enjoyment and Digestive Well-Being

Beyond their health benefits, the diverse flavors and textures of living foods enhance the culinary experience, promoting mindful and enjoyable eating.

A positive relationship with food can contribute to overall digestive well-being.

In the grand tapestry of health, the impact of living foods on digestion weaves a narrative of enzymatic brilliance, microbial harmony, and nutrient-rich sustenance. From the vibrant crunch of raw vegetables to the probiotic embrace of fermented delights, living foods unfold as allies in the intricate dance of digestion, nurturing the body and fostering a state of holistic well-being.

Enhanced Energy Levels

Embark on a thorough exploration of the invigorating effects that living foods impart on the body, unraveling the intricate mechanisms through which these vibrant edibles elevate energy levels and contribute to a dynamic sense of well-being.

Nutrient Density

Living foods, such as raw fruits, vegetables, and sprouts, are nutrient-dense, providing a spectrum of vitamins, minerals, and antioxidants.

This nutritional richness fuels the body with essential elements, fostering optimal energy metabolism.

Enzymatic Activation

The enzymes present in living foods play a pivotal role in breaking down nutrients and facilitating their absorption.

Enhanced enzymatic activity contributes to efficient energy extraction from food.

Natural Hydration

Many living foods have a high water content, contributing to hydration.

Proper hydration is fundamental for cellular functions and energy production within the body.

Balancing Macronutrients

Living foods often offer a balanced mix of macronutrients—carbohydrates, proteins, and healthy fats.

This balance provides a sustained release of energy throughout the day.

Blood Sugar Regulation

The fiber in living foods helps regulate blood sugar levels.

Stable blood sugar levels contribute to sustained energy, preventing the highs and lows associated with refined sugars.

Mitochondrial Support

Antioxidants in living foods protect cellular structures, including mitochondria—the energy-producing powerhouses of cells.

This protection supports efficient energy production and helps combat oxidative stress.

B Vitamins and Energy Metabolism

Living foods are rich in B vitamins, crucial for energy metabolism.

B vitamins participate in converting food into energy and are integral to the proper functioning of the nervous system.

Adaptogens and Stress Response

Certain living foods, such as adaptogenic herbs, may support the body's response to stress.

Improved stress management contributes to sustained energy levels.

Oxygenation and Alkalinity

Living foods contribute to an alkaline environment in the body.

An alkaline state supports efficient oxygenation of tissues, a key factor in energy production.

Probiotics and Gut-Brain Connection

Fermented living foods introduce beneficial probiotics to the gut.

The gut-brain connection influences energy levels, mood, and cognitive function, highlighting the holistic impact of living foods.

Hygiene of Living Foods

Living foods, consumed in their raw and unprocessed state, preserve their inherent vitality.

The hygiene of these foods ensures that their nutritional potency remains intact, contributing to sustained energy.

Mindful Eating and Energy

The act of consuming living foods mindfully fosters a positive relationship with food. Mindful eating practices can enhance satisfaction and promote a more sustained and balanced energy release.

In the intricate dance of nutrition, living foods emerge as catalysts for vitality, infusing the body with a symphony of nutrients and a burst of life force. From enzymatic prowess to the balancing act of macronutrients, these edibles contribute to a dynamic interplay that fuels the body, supporting enhanced energy levels and fostering a vibrant state of well-being.

Potential disease prevention

Embark on a comprehensive journey through the potential disease-preventive aspects of consuming living foods, unraveling the intricate ways in which these vibrant edibles may contribute to a resilient shield against various health challenges.

Antioxidant Armory

Living foods, rich in antioxidants, act as a formidable defense against oxidative stress. Antioxidants neutralize free radicals, reducing the risk of cellular damage linked to chronic diseases.

Immune Boosting Nutrients

Nutrient-dense living foods provide essential vitamins and minerals vital for a robust immune system.

A well-nourished immune system is better equipped to fend off infections and prevent illness.

Inflammation Management

Many living foods possess anti-inflammatory properties, helping to modulate chronic inflammation—a common factor in various diseases.

A diet rich in anti-inflammatory foods may contribute to long-term disease prevention.

Gut Microbiome Harmony

Probiotics in fermented living foods support a balanced gut microbiome.

A healthy microbiome is associated with a lower risk of gastrointestinal issues, autoimmune conditions, and metabolic diseases.

Blood Sugar Regulation

Living foods, particularly those high in fiber, aid in regulating blood sugar levels.

Stable blood sugar is crucial in preventing type 2 diabetes and reducing the risk of heart disease.

Heart Health Support

Living foods contribute to heart health by promoting healthy blood pressure, reducing cholesterol levels, and preventing arterial plaque formation.

Omega-3 fatty acids in certain living foods offer additional cardiovascular benefits.

Cancer Protective Compounds

Phytonutrients and bioactive compounds in living foods exhibit potential anti-cancer properties.

Regular consumption may contribute to preventing certain types of cancers.

Bone Health Nutrients

Living foods rich in calcium, magnesium, and vitamin K support bone health.

Adequate intake of these nutrients may reduce the risk of osteoporosis and fractures.

Hormonal Balance

Living foods contribute to hormonal balance through their diverse nutrient profile.

Balanced hormones play a role in preventing conditions such as hormonal cancers and reproductive issues.

Disease-Fighting Enzymes

Enzymes in living foods contribute to digestion and metabolic processes.

Proper enzyme function may play a role in preventing diseases related to impaired digestion and nutrient absorption.

Hydration and Kidney Health

Living foods with high water content contribute to hydration.

Adequate hydration supports kidney function, reducing the risk of kidney-related diseases.

Mental Health Connection

The gut-brain axis influenced by living foods may contribute to mental health.

A healthy gut is linked to a lower risk of mental health disorders and neurodegenerative diseases.

Lifestyle Impact

Embracing a diet rich in living foods often correlates with a health-conscious lifestyle.

Combined with other healthy habits, living foods contribute to a holistic approach to disease prevention.

In the tapestry of health, living foods emerge as a potent ally, weaving a narrative of disease prevention through a myriad of nutritional and protective mechanisms. From antioxidant prowess to immune fortification, these vibrant edibles stand as a cornerstone in fostering a resilient shield against the complex landscape of health challenges.

Chapter 5 Preparing Living Food.

Raw Food Preparation Techniques

Enter the culinary realm where creativity dances with simplicity—raw food preparation, an art form that celebrates the unadulterated beauty of nature's bounty. Picture a kitchen as a canvas, and each raw ingredient as a stroke of vibrant color, waiting to compose a masterpiece of flavors, textures, and nutritional wonders.

Culinary Choreography

Raw food preparation is a choreography of techniques that respect the essence of ingredients.

Knife skills become a dance, transforming crisp vegetables and juicy fruits into edible works of art.

Marination Magic

Marinating raw foods introduces flavors that tango with the taste buds.

Citrus-infused marinades and herb dances elevate the freshness of raw ingredients to a crescendo of taste.

Delectable Dehydration

Dehydrating fruits and vegetables is like capturing the essence of sunshine.

- This technique intensifies flavors, creating nature's candy without compromising vitality.

Spiralized Symphony

Spiraled vegetable twirl on the plate, creating a visual and textural spectacle.

Zucchini and carrots become the prima ballerinas, ready to delight in a crisp and colorful pas de deux.

Nut Milk Ballet

Crafting nut milk transforms raw nuts into a creamy ballet of richness.

Almonds, cashews, or macadamias pirouette into silky elixirs, ready to enchant in smoothies and desserts.

Avocado Artistry

Avocado, the velvety muse of raw cuisine, takes center stage.

Mashed, sliced, or elegantly fanned, it adds a buttery touch to salads, wraps, and raw sushi creations.

Vibrant Ceviche

Raw fish, marinated in citrus, becomes a lively Latin dance on the palate.

Ceviche showcases the beauty of simplicity, allowing the natural flavors to shine.

Sprout Ballet

Sprouting seeds and legumes is a ballet of life unfolding.

Tiny sprouts pirouette into salads, wraps, and sandwiches, bringing a burst of vitality to every bite.

Raw Chocolate Elegance

Raw cacao, the dark star of raw desserts, orchestrates a symphony of richness.

Nut and date confections become the canvas for a chocolate masterpiece, guilt-free and indulgent.

Floral Infusions

Edible flowers, delicate and vibrant, weave through salads and desserts.

The culinary ballet is elevated with floral notes, creating a sensory experience that transcends taste.

Minimalist Plating

Raw food presentation is a study of minimalist elegance.

Each plate is a canvas, allowing the natural colors and textures to tell a story of freshness and vitality.

Fermentation Waltz

Fermented creations perform a waltz of flavors and gut health benefits.

Kimchi, sauerkraut, and pickles dance with tangy notes, enriching the palate and supporting digestion.

In the enchanting world of raw food preparation, the kitchen becomes a stage, and every technique is a choreographed movement in a dance of flavors. It's a celebration where ingredients shine in their purest form, inviting you to partake in the artistry of raw culinary creativity.

Tips for Incorporating Living Foods

Step into the vibrant tapestry of nutrition, where living foods beckon with their vitality and flavors. Here are tips that transform your culinary journey into a celebration of life through the art of incorporating living foods:

Embrace the Rainbow

Paint your plate with a spectrum of colors. Each hue represents different nutrients and antioxidants found in fruits, vegetables, and sprouts.

Fresh and Local Dance

Let the seasons guide your choices. Local, seasonal produce not only bursts with flavor but also ensures optimal freshness and nutritional content.

Culinary Alchemy with Sprouts

Elevate your salads, wraps, and sandwiches with the magic of sprouts. These tiny powerhouses add a crunch of life and a burst of nutrients.

Ferment for Flavor

Dive into the world of fermentation. Experiment with kimchi, sauerkraut, or kombucha to introduce lively, probiotic-rich flavors to your meals.

Unleash the Nut Milk Symphony

Discover the art of crafting your nut milk. Almonds, cashews, or hazelnuts can be the stars of your creamy elixirs, enriching smoothies and desserts.

Garden-to-Table Bliss

Cultivate a small herb garden. Fresh herbs like basil, cilantro, and mint are not just aromatic; they infuse living foods with a burst of freshness.

The Raw Dessert Ballet

Indulge in the sweet side of living foods. Raw desserts, sweetened with natural sources like dates and fruits, offer guilt-free indulgence.

Mindful Meal Prep Meditation

Engage in mindful meal preparation. The act of chopping, slicing, and arranging becomes a meditation, infusing your dishes with positive energy.

Avocado Elegance

Avocado, the creamy virtuoso, can be your culinary companion. Mash it for spreads, slice it for salads, or enjoy it as a standalone delight.

Play with Texture

Experiment with textures. Mix crunchy nuts with silky smooth avocados, or pair juicy fruits with crisp vegetables for a delightful mouthfeel.

Fusion of Flavors

Embrace flavor fusion. Mix and match herbs, spices, and condiments to create a symphony of tastes that dance on your taste buds.

Culinary Artistry with Edible Flowers

Elevate your presentations with edible flowers. Their delicate beauty adds a touch of elegance and a hint of floral notes to your dishes.

Savor the Simplicity

Appreciate the simplicity of living foods. Sometimes, the most delightful dishes are born from a handful of fresh, unprocessed ingredients.

In the culinary ballet of living foods, your kitchen transforms into a stage for nutritional artistry. These tips invite you to dance with flavors, colors, and textures, creating a symphony of living foods that nourish not only your body but also your spirit.

Chapter 6 Common Misconceptions

Addressing Concerns About Safety

Navigating the realm of living foods is an exciting culinary journey, but it's essential to address concerns about safety to ensure a wholesome and risk-free experience. Let's explore these considerations in detail:

1. Microbial Safety in Sprouts

Concern: Sprouts, particularly alfalfa and mung bean sprouts, are associated with foodborne illnesses due to bacterial contamination.

Safety Measures: Thoroughly rinse and sanitize sprouting equipment. Choose reputable sources for sprouting seeds, and ensure proper hygiene during the sprouting process.

2. Bacterial Risks in Fermentation

Concern: Fermented foods, like kimchi or sauerkraut, are prone to contamination by harmful bacteria.

Safety Measures: Use clean utensils and containers. Submerge ingredients in brine to create an anaerobic environment that inhibits harmful bacteria. Ferment in a controlled environment and follow established recipes.

3. Allergen Cross-Contamination

Concern: Cross-contamination can occur when preparing living foods, especially if there are allergens in the kitchen.

Safety Measures: Clean utensils, cutting boards, and surfaces thoroughly between different foods. Designate specific tools for living foods to prevent cross-contamination.

4. Parasitic Concerns in Raw Fish

Concern: Consuming raw fish, as in sushi, may pose risks of parasitic infections.

Safety Measures: Source high-quality, sushi-grade fish from reputable suppliers. Freeze fish at appropriate temperatures to kill potential parasites.

5. Risk of Food Poisoning in Raw Meats

<u>Concern</u>: Consuming raw meats, like beef tartare, carries a risk of foodborne pathogens.

<u>Safety Measures</u>: Purchase high-quality, fresh meats from trusted sources. Adhere to strict hygiene practices during handling and preparation.

6. Contamination in Raw Dairy

<u>Concern</u>: Raw milk and dairy products can harbor harmful bacteria such as E. coli or Salmonella.

<u>Safety Measures</u>: Choose pasteurized dairy to eliminate the risk of harmful bacteria. If consuming raw dairy, ensure it

comes from a reputable source adhering to strict safety standards.

7. Proper Handling of Raw Eggs

<u>Concern</u>: Raw eggs in dishes like Caesar salad dressing may pose a risk of Salmonella contamination.

<u>Safety Measures</u>: Use pasteurized eggs when consuming raw or undercooked dishes. Store eggs properly and be cautious with dishes containing raw eggs, especially for vulnerable populations.

8. Hygiene in Living Food Preparation

<u>Concern</u>: General concerns about hygiene during the preparation of living foods.

<u>Safety Measures</u>: Wash hands thoroughly before handling living foods. Clean all

utensils, cutting boards, and surfaces meticulously. Follow proper food safety guidelines.

9. Mold Contamination in Fermented Foods

<u>Concern</u>: Improper fermentation conditions may lead to mold growth.

<u>Safety Measures</u>: Use clean, airtight containers for fermentation. Discard any batch showing signs of mold. Follow recommended fermentation times and conditions.

10. Individual Sensitivities

<u>Concern</u>: Some individuals may have specific sensitivities or allergies to certain living foods.

<u>Safety Measures</u>: Be aware of individual sensitivities and allergies. Introduce new living foods gradually to monitor any adverse reactions.

Navigating the world of living foods with safety in mind ensures a delightful and risk-free experience. By incorporating these safety measures, enthusiasts can savor the benefits of living foods while minimizing potential concerns.

Balancing a Living Foods Diet

Embark on a culinary odyssey, where the vibrant harmony of flavors and the nutritional symphony dance in tandem—a journey of balancing a living foods diet, where freshness meets fulfillment. Picture your plate as a canvas, and each living food ingredient as a brushstroke, creating a masterpiece of vitality and balance.

1. The Palette of Colors

   - Envision your plate as a palette of colors, each hue representing a spectrum of nutrients. From the deep greens of kale to the fiery reds of bell peppers, let diversity be your guiding principle.

2. Nature's Symphony of Textures

   - Explore the rich tapestry of textures nature offers. The crispness of fresh vegetables, the creaminess of avocados, and the crunch of nuts—let your bites compose a symphony of sensations.

3. Leafy Greens Ballet

Let leafy greens take center stage. Spinach, kale, and arugula pirouette onto your plate, bringing a burst of vitamins, minerals, and chlorophyll—the essence of plant vitality.

4. Proteins in a Dance of Variety

Embrace a diverse array of proteins. From the grace of legumes to the elegance of nuts and seeds, let protein sources waltz through your meals, offering a complete amino acid profile.

5. Fermentation's Tangy Tango:

Invite the tangy allure of fermented foods to join the dance. Kimchi, sauerkraut, and kombucha add a lively note, supporting gut health and introducing a flavorful twist.

6. Sprouting Elegance:

Sprouts, the tiny dancers of the living foods stage, infuse your meals with youthful vigor. Sprinkle them atop salads and wraps, letting their freshness elevate your culinary experience.

7. Fruits in a Sweet Serenade

Let fruits serenade your taste buds with natural sweetness. Berries, citrus, and tropical delights bring a fruity crescendo to your living foods repertoire.

8. Hydration Ballet

Hydration, a graceful ballet in the background, is essential. Infuse your meals with hydrating fruits and vegetables, ensuring your body dances through each day with vitality.

9. Mindful Eating Waltz:

Engage in the mindful eating waltz. Slow down, savor each bite, and let the flavors unfold like a dance, fostering a deeper connection with your nourishment.

10. The Probiotic Pas de Deux

Allow probiotics to perform a pas de deux in your gut. Yogurt, kefir, and other fermented dairy or plant-based options harmonize with your digestive system, promoting balance.

11. Nuts and Seeds Ballet

Nuts and seeds, the versatile dancers, add a touch of decadence. From the creamy elegance of almond butter to the crunch of chia seeds, let them pirouette through your recipes.

12. Culinary Improvisation:

Embrace the spirit of culinary improvisation. Let your creativity sway with the seasons, exploring local, fresh produce and discovering new ways to compose your living foods symphony.

In the artful dance of balancing a living food diet, your culinary choices become the choreography of well-being. With each bite, you not only savor flavors but also conduct a nourishing symphony that celebrates the vitality of life on your plate.

Chapter 7　　Recipes

Simple Living Foods Recipes

Embark on a culinary journey where simplicity harmonizes with nourishment—a collection of simple living foods recipes that celebrate the vibrant essence of fresh, unprocessed ingredients. These recipes unfold as a culinary sonnet, inviting you to embrace the art of simplicity in your kitchen.

1. Garden Fresh Salad Symphony

     Ingredients:

   - Mixed greens (kale, spinach, arugula)
   - Cherry tomatoes
   - Cucumber

- Avocado
- Red onion
   Dressing:
- Olive oil
- Balsamic vinegar
- Dijon mustard
- Salt and pepper
   Method:
- Toss the crisp greens with colorful
   vegetables.
- Whisk together the dressing ingredients
   and drizzle over the salad.
- A refreshing ode to the garden on your
   plate.

2. Mango Avocado Salsa Serenade
   Ingredients:
- Ripe mango

- Avocado

- Red onion

- Fresh cilantro

- Lime juice

  Method:

- Dice mango and avocado into bite-sized

  pieces.

  - Finely chop red onion and cilantro.

- Mix ingredients and squeeze fresh lime

  juice.

  - A tropical salsa that dances with

  sweetness and zest.

3. Quinoa Buddha Bowl Ballet

  Ingredients:

- Cooked quinoa

- Steamed broccoli

- Sliced radishes

- Shredded carrots

- Chickpeas (roasted)

- Sauce:

- Tahini

- Lemon juice

- Garlic

- Water (to adjust consistency)

  Method:

- Assemble quinoa, vegetables, and

  chickpeas in a bowl.

- Drizzle with creamy tahini sauce.

- A nourishing bowl that pirouettes with

  plant-based goodness.

4. Zucchini Noodles Pas de Deux

   Ingredients:

   - Zucchini (spiralized)

   - Cherry tomatoes

- Pesto sauce

- Pine nuts

  Method:

- Spiralize zucchini into noodles.

- Toss with halved cherry tomatoes.

- Coat with vibrant pesto and sprinkle
  pine nuts.

- A low-carb symphony of flavors and
  textures.

5. Berry Coconut Chia Pudding Sonata
   Ingredients:
   - Chia seeds

   - Coconut milk

   - Mixed berries (strawberries, blueberries)

   - Maple syrup

Method:

- Mix chia seeds with coconut milk and let
  it is set.

- Layer with fresh berries and a drizzle of
  maple syrup.

- A sweet, nutritious melody in every
  spoonful.

6. Refreshing Cucumber Mint Cooler Waltz
    Ingredients:

- Cucumber slices

- Fresh mint leaves

- Lemon slices

- Sparkling water
  Method:

- Combine cucumber, mint, and lemon in
  a glass.

- Top with sparkling water.

- A crisp and revitalizing dance for your taste buds.

7. Avocado Chocolate Mousse Rhapsody
    - Ingredients:
    - Ripe avocados
    - Cocoa powder
    - Maple syrup
    - Vanilla extract
      Method:
    - Blend avocados, cocoa powder, maple syrup, and vanilla until smooth.
    - Chill and serve.
    - A velvety, guilt-free indulgence for the sweet tooth.

8. Sesame Ginger Tofu Stir-Fry Minuet
    Ingredients:

- Tofu cubes

- Mixed vegetables (bell peppers, broccoli, snow peas)

- Soy sauce

- Sesame oil

- Ginger and garlic (minced)
  Method:

- Sauté tofu until golden, then add vegetables.

- Stir in soy sauce, sesame oil, ginger, and garlic.

- A savory stir-fry that twirls with Asian-inspired flavors.

In the realm of simple living food recipes, these culinary compositions celebrate the elegance of minimalism, allowing the freshness and flavors of each ingredient to shine in a gastronomic symphony. Let simplicity be your culinary muse as you dance through these nourishing and delightful recipes.

Meal Ideas for a Balanced Living Foods Diet

Here's a collection of meal ideas that seamlessly weave together the vibrancy of living foods into a symphony of flavors and nutrients.

Morning Radiance Smoothie
  - Ingredients:
  - Kale leaves
  - Banana

- Mixed berries (blueberries,
   strawberries)
- Chia seeds
- Coconut water
   Method:
- Blend kale, banana, berries, chia seeds,
   and coconut water.
- A vibrant green elixir that kickstarts
   your day with energy and antioxidants.

2. Sunrise Acai Bowl Ballet
   - Ingredients:
   - Acai puree
   - Granola
   - Sliced kiwi, mango, and berries
   - Coconut flakes
   - Almond butter drizzle

Method:

- Top acai puree with granola, fresh fruits, coconut flakes, and a swirl of almond butter.
- A visually stunning bowl that dances with varied textures and flavors.

3. Quinoa Power Salad Overture

   - Ingredients:
   - Quinoa (cooked)
   - Spinach
   - Cherry tomatoes
   - Avocado
   - Chickpeas (roasted)
   - Lemon-tahini dressing

   Method:

   - Combine quinoa, spinach, tomatoes, avocado, and roasted chickpeas.
   - Drizzle with a zesty lemon-tahini

dressing.

- A nutrient-packed ensemble that satisfies and energizes.

4. Crisp Nori Wrap Waltz

   Ingredients:

   - Nori sheets

   - Jicama noodles

   - Carrot ribbons

   - Cucumber strips

   - Avocado slices

   - Sesame ginger dressing

   Method:

   - Assemble jicama, carrot, cucumber, and avocado in nori sheets.

   - Drizzle with sesame ginger dressing.

   - A refreshing dance of colors and crunch.

5. Miso-Glazed Tempeh Tango

Ingredients:

- Tempeh slices

- Broccoli florets

- Quinoa

- Miso glaze

- Sesame seeds

Method:

- Sauté tempeh and broccoli, then toss with quinoa.

- Glaze with miso dressing and sprinkle sesame seeds.

- A savory performance that marries protein and plant goodness.

6. Zesty Cauliflower Rice Samba

Ingredients:

- Cauliflower rice
- Bell peppers
- Black beans
- Corn kernels
- Fresh cilantro
- Lime wedges
  Method:
- Sauté cauliflower rice with bell peppers,
  black beans, and corn.
- Garnish with cilantro and serve with
  lime wedges.
- A lively, low-carb dance that bursts with
  Mexican-inspired flavors.

7. Dazzling Fruit Sushi Finale
   Ingredients:
- Nori sheets
- Sliced mango, kiwi, and strawberries

- Coconut rice

- Almond butter drizzle

  Method:

- Spread coconut rice on nori sheets and add sliced fruits.

- Roll and slice into bite-sized pieces.

- A sweet, sushi-inspired creation that brings a delightful closure to your day.

In this culinary spectacle of balanced living foods, each meal is an invitation to savor the freshness, colors, and textures that nature offers. Let these meal ideas be your inspiration as you choreograph a daily gastronomic symphony that nourishes both body and soul.

Chapter 8 Conclusion

Summary of Benefits

Embrace the vitality of living foods and unlock a myriad of benefits that contribute to your overall well-being:

Nutrient Density: Living foods are rich in vitamins, minerals, and antioxidants, providing a potent dose of essential nutrients.

Enzymatic Power: Enzymes present in living foods support digestion, nutrient absorption, and overall metabolic processes.

Hydration and Fiber: Many living foods have high water content, contributing to hydration, while their fiber content aids digestion and promotes satiety.

Balanced Macronutrients: Living foods offer a harmonious mix of carbohydrates, proteins, and healthy fats, supporting a balanced diet.

Blood Sugar Regulation: Fiber in living foods helps stabilize blood sugar levels, reducing the risk of diabetes and promoting sustained energy.

Heart Health Support: Living foods contribute to cardiovascular health by regulating blood pressure, reducing cholesterol, and supporting overall heart function.

Antioxidant Defense: Abundant in antioxidants, living foods combat oxidative stress, reducing the risk of cellular damage and chronic diseases.

Gut Microbiome Harmony: Fermented living foods introduce beneficial probiotics, promoting a healthy gut microbiome and supporting digestive health.

Bone Health Nutrients: Living foods rich in calcium, magnesium, and vitamin K contribute to strong and healthy bones, reducing the risk of osteoporosis.

Hormonal Balance: The diverse nutrient profile of living foods supports hormonal balance, influencing various aspects of health, including reproductive health and cancer prevention.

Mental Well-being: The gut-brain connection influenced by living foods may contribute to mental health, fostering a positive impact on mood and cognitive function.

Improved Digestion: Enzymes and probiotics in living foods support efficient digestion, reducing bloating, gas, and other digestive issues.

Enhanced Energy Levels: Living foods provide sustained energy through nutrient-dense sources, balanced macronutrients, and efficient energy metabolism.

Disease Prevention: The antioxidant, anti-inflammatory, and immune-boosting properties of living foods contribute to the prevention of various diseases.

Hygiene and Safety: Proper handling and preparation of living foods minimize the risk of contamination, ensuring a safe and wholesome culinary experience.

Incorporating living foods into your diet can be a delicious and holistic approach to promoting health, vitality, and a profound sense of well-being.

Encouragement for Adoption

Here's a heartfelt encouragement to inspire the adoption of these nourishing delights into your daily life. Embark on a journey of well-being as you consider the vibrant embrace of living foods:

1. Embrace Nature's Bounty

   - Dive into a world where the colors, flavors, and textures of fresh, living foods become your culinary canvas. Nature's bounty awaits, offering a palette of vitality to elevate your dining experience.

2. Nourish with Vibrancy

Picture your plate as a celebration of life—bursting with vibrant greens, rich reds, and the sun-kissed hues of fresh fruits. Embrace living foods as the essence of nutrition, nourishing not just your body but your spirit.

3. Savor the Symphony of Flavors

Delight in the symphony of flavors that living foods offer. From the crisp crunch of vegetables to the juicy burst of fruits, each bite is a melody, inviting you to savor the richness of unprocessed goodness.

4. Energize Your Essence

Feel the surge of energy that accompanies every bite. Living foods are a powerhouse of nutrients, infusing your body with vitality, supporting optimal health, and enhancing your zest for life.

5. Nurture Your Inner Garden

Imagine your body as a garden, and living foods as the seeds that nurture your inner sanctuary. Cultivate health and well-being as you tend to this garden with the wholesome, unprocessed gifts that nature provides.

6. Sustainable Wellness Journey

View the adoption of living foods as a sustainable wellness journey. It's not just a diet; it's a lifestyle that harmonizes with the rhythms of nature, fostering a sense of balance, mindfulness, and enduring well-being.

7. Connect with Your Culinary Roots

Reconnect with the simplicity of your culinary roots. Living foods bring you back to the basics, celebrating the purity of ingredients and honoring the age-old wisdom of nourishing the body with what nature provides.

8. Listen to Your Body's Symphony

Pay attention to the subtle symphony your body orchestrates in response to living foods. Feel the surge of energy, the clarity of mind, and the gentle well-being that accompanies a diet rich in freshness and life force.

9. Sustainable Earth, Sustainable You

Acknowledge the interconnectedness of a diet centered around living foods with the well-being of the planet. By choosing unprocessed, plant-based options, you contribute not only to your health but also to the sustainability of the Earth.

10. Celebrate Your Wellness Journey

Every meal is a celebration of your wellness journey. Whether it's a simple salad or a gourmet living foods creation, relish each bite as a testament to your commitment to a nourished and vibrant life.

In the tapestry of well-being, the adoption of living foods is an invitation to celebrate the beauty of simplicity, the richness of nature's offerings, and the vibrant symphony that nourishes not just the body but the essence of who you are. Let the journey unfold with joy, curiosity, and the unwavering belief that you are sowing the seeds of a healthier, more vibrant you.

www.ingramcontent.com/pod-product-compliance
Lightning Source LLC
Chambersburg PA
CBHW070911260726
48661CB00004B/1691